JAXON SKYE

Screen Serenity

Balancing Mental Health in a Connected World

First edition

This book was professionally typeset on Reedsy.
Find out more at reedsy.com

Contents

1

Introduction

Overview

In an era where digital devices dominate our daily lives, achieving a state of "Screen Serenity" is more critical than ever. This book explores the impact of digital technology on mental health and provides practical strategies for maintaining a healthy balance between our online and offline worlds. By understanding the benefits and drawbacks of our connected world, we can better navigate the complexities of modern life and foster a healthier relationship with technology.

The Digital Age

The digital age has transformed how we communicate, work, and entertain ourselves. With the rise of smartphones, social media, and instant access to information, we are more connected than ever before. While these advancements bring numerous benefits, they also present significant challenges to our mental health. This book aims to shed light on these challenges and offer solutions to achieve a balanced and serene digital life.

Chapter 1: The Impact of Digital Technology on Mental Health

In the contemporary era, digital technology has revolutionized the way we communicate, work, and interact with the world around us. At the forefront of this technological revolution are digital devices such as smartphones, tablets, and computers, along with the vast array of applications and platforms they offer. These tools have undeniably brought numerous benefits to our lives, facilitating instant communication with loved ones across the globe, providing access to an endless trove of information, and offering avenues for social connection and support. The ability to stay connected with friends and family, regardless of geographical distance, has transformed the way we maintain relationships, fostering a sense of closeness and intimacy that transcends physical boundaries. Moreover, the internet serves as a vast repository of knowledge, with a wealth of resources readily available at our fingertips. From online courses and tutorials to educational websites and research databases, digital technology has democratized access to information, empowering individuals to pursue lifelong learning and personal growth. Additionally, digital platforms have emerged as invaluable resources for mental health support, offering online therapy services, support groups, and mental wellness apps designed to promote emotional well-being and resilience.

However, alongside these undeniable benefits, the pervasive influence of digital technology has also given rise to significant challenges and concerns regarding its impact on mental health. One such concern is the prevalence of social media and its role in shaping our perceptions of self and others. Social media platforms, such as Facebook, Instagram, and Twitter, have become integral parts of daily life for millions of people worldwide, offering spaces for social connection, self-expression, and community building. Yet, the curated nature of social media content often presents an idealized version of reality, where users showcase their happiest moments and most flattering angles, creating a distorted image of what constitutes a "perfect" life. This phenomenon can lead to feelings of inadequacy and self-doubt as individuals compare their own lives to the carefully curated highlight reels of others, fostering a culture of comparison and competition that can erode self-esteem and contribute to negative mental health outcomes.

Moreover, the constant exposure to digital technology and the relentless stream of information it provides can lead to a phenomenon known as "information overload," where individuals feel overwhelmed by the sheer volume of content available to them. This constant barrage of stimuli can lead to heightened levels of stress, anxiety, and cognitive fatigue as individuals struggle to process and make sense of the vast amount of information vying for their attention. Additionally, the pressure to stay connected and responsive in an increasingly interconnected world can create a sense of digital fatigue, where individuals feel exhausted and burnt out from the constant demands of technology.

Furthermore, the anonymity and disinhibition afforded by digital platforms can give rise to a range of harmful behaviors, including cyber-bullying and online harassment, which can have devastating consequences for mental health. The impersonal nature of online interactions can embolden individuals to engage in behaviors they would not otherwise exhibit in face-to-face settings, leading to a culture of toxicity and negativity that can be deeply damaging to those on the receiving end. Additionally, the omnipresence of digital devices and the constant connectivity they afford can disrupt our natural sleep-wake cycles, leading to sleep disturbances and fatigue that can further exacerbate mental health issues.

Chapter 2: Understanding Digital Addiction

In the digital age, the phenomenon of digital addiction has emerged as a significant concern, drawing attention to the compulsive use of digital devices and the internet at the expense of other aspects of life. Digital addiction encompasses a spectrum of behaviors, ranging from excessive use of social media and gaming to compulsive web surfing and online shopping, all of which can have profound implications for mental health and well-being. At its core, digital addiction shares many similarities with traditional forms of addiction, driven by underlying psychological mechanisms that reinforce and perpetuate compulsive behaviors. One such mechanism is the brain's reward system, which is activated in response to pleasurable stimuli and plays a central role in shaping our behavior and decision-making processes. When we engage in activities that elicit a sense of pleasure or reward, such as receiving likes on a social media post or winning a game, our brain releases dopamine, a neurotransmitter associated with feelings of pleasure and satisfaction. Over time, repeated exposure to these rewarding stimuli can lead to desensitization, where the brain's reward system becomes less responsive to natural rewards, such as spending time with loved ones or engaging in hobbies, and more reliant on the artificial rewards provided by digital devices and online activities.

Additionally, the design of digital applications and platforms plays a crucial role in shaping user behavior and fostering addictive patterns of use. Many digital products are designed with features such as infinite scrolling, notifications, and personalized recommendations, all of which are intended to maximize user engagement and keep users coming back for more. These design choices are often informed by principles of behavioral psychology, such as variable reinforcement schedules and the scarcity effect, which exploit cognitive biases and psychological vulnerabilities to encourage repeated engagement. For example, the intermittent rewards provided by social media platforms, such as likes, comments, and shares, create a sense of unpredictability and anticipation that can keep users hooked, while the fear of missing out (FOMO) motivates individuals to constantly check their devices for updates and notifications.

Recognizing digital addiction requires an understanding of its signs and symptoms, which can manifest in various ways depending on the individual and the nature of their digital habits. Common signs of digital addiction include spending excessive amounts of time on digital devices, experiencing withdrawal symptoms when unable to access digital technology, neglecting responsibilities and obligations in favor of digital activities, and using digital devices as a primary means of coping with stress or negative emotions. Additionally, individuals with digital addiction may exhibit changes in mood and behavior, such as irritability, anxiety, or depression, as well as physical symptoms such as headaches, eye strain, and disrupted sleep patterns. It is important to note that digital addiction is not limited to a specific age group or demographic; people of all ages can be affected by digital addiction, from teenagers who spend hours scrolling through social media to adults who find themselves unable to disconnect from work emails and notifications.

Addressing digital addiction requires a multifaceted approach that addresses both individual and systemic factors contributing to problematic digital use. On an individual level, strategies such as setting limits on screen time, practicing mindfulness and self-awareness, and seeking support from friends, family, or mental health professionals can be effective in managing digital addiction. Additionally, fostering a culture of digital wellness in homes, schools, and workplaces can help promote healthy digital habits and mitigate the risk of digital addiction. This includes educating individuals about the potential risks of excessive digital use, providing resources and support for those struggling with digital addiction, and creating environments that prioritize well-being and balance in all aspects of life. By raising awareness of digital addiction and empowering individuals to take control of their digital habits, we can work towards a healthier and more balanced relationship with digital technology in the modern age.

Chapter 3: The Effects of Screen Time on Mental Health

In the digital age, screen time—the amount of time spent using digital devices such as smartphones, tablets, computers, and televisions—has become a significant factor in shaping our mental health and well-being. While digital technology offers numerous benefits, including instant access to information, communication with others, and entertainment, excessive screen time can have detrimental effects on our mental health. One area where the effects of screen time are particularly pronounced is in its impact on physical and mental health. Research has shown that prolonged screen time can disrupt our natural sleep-wake cycle, leading to sleep disturbances and poor sleep quality. The blue light emitted by screens interferes with the production of melatonin, a hormone that regulates sleep, making it harder to fall asleep and stay asleep at night. As a result, individuals who spend excessive amounts of time on digital devices may experience insomnia, fatigue, and daytime sleepiness, all of which can impair cognitive function, mood, and overall well-being.

Moreover, excessive screen time has been linked to a range of emotional and psychological issues, including anxiety, depression, and stress. The constant exposure to social media, news, and other digital content can create a constant barrage of stimuli that overwhelms our cognitive capacities and triggers feelings of anxiety and agitation. Social media, in particular, has been implicated in the exacerbation of mental health issues, with studies linking heavy social media use to increased levels of depression, loneliness, and social isolation. The curated nature of social media content, where users often present an idealized version of themselves and their lives, can lead to feelings of inadequacy and low self-esteem as individuals compare themselves unfavorably to others. Additionally, the constant stream of negative news and information on digital platforms can contribute to feelings of stress and anxiety, as individuals struggle to make sense of and process the overwhelming amount of information bombarding them on a daily basis.

Cognitive effects are another significant aspect of screen time's impact on mental health. Excessive screen time has been shown to impair cognitive functions such as attention, concentration, and memory, leading to reduced academic performance and impaired cognitive development, particularly in children and adolescents. The constant multitasking and switching between screens and tasks can overload our cognitive resources, making it difficult to focus and concentrate on any one task for an extended period. This fragmented attention can have long-term consequences for our ability to learn, retain information, and problem-solve, as our brains become accustomed to constant stimulation and instant gratification provided by digital devices.

Furthermore, the sedentary nature of screen time can contribute to physical health issues such as obesity, cardiovascular disease, and musculoskeletal problems. Spending long hours sitting in front of a screen can lead to a sedentary lifestyle, where individuals engage in minimal physical activity and spend the majority of their day in a seated position. This lack of physical activity not only increases the risk of chronic health conditions but also has implications for mental health, as regular exercise has been shown to improve mood, reduce stress, and enhance cognitive function. Additionally, the posture adopted while using digital devices, such as slouching or hunching over, can contribute to musculoskeletal issues such as neck and back pain, further exacerbating physical discomfort and reducing overall well-being.

In conclusion, while digital technology offers numerous benefits, excessive screen time can have significant implications for our mental and physical health. By understanding the effects of screen time on mental health, we can take steps to mitigate its negative impact and foster a healthier relationship with digital devices. This includes setting limits on screen time, practicing mindfulness and self-awareness, and incorporating regular breaks and physical activity into our daily routines. By prioritizing our mental and physical well-being, we can ensure that screen time enhances rather than detracts from our quality of life in the digital age.

5

Chapter 4: Strategies for Managing Screen Time

In the digital age, managing screen time has become increasingly important for maintaining mental health and well-being. Excessive screen time has been associated with a range of negative outcomes, including sleep disturbances, anxiety, depression, and cognitive impairments. Therefore, developing effective strategies for managing screen time is essential for promoting a healthy balance between digital technology and other aspects of life. One key strategy for managing screen time is setting boundaries and limits on the amount of time spent using digital devices. This can involve establishing specific time limits for different activities, such as checking email or social media, as well as designating screen-free times and areas, such as during meals or before bedtime. By setting clear boundaries around screen time, individuals can reduce the risk of excessive use and create space for other activities and interests.

Another important strategy for managing screen time is practicing mindful technology use. This involves being intentional and aware of how and why we use digital devices, as well as the impact they have on our mental and emotional well-being. Mindful technology use can include techniques such as taking regular breaks from screens, limiting multitasking, and engaging fully in offline activities. By cultivating mindfulness in our interactions with technology, we can become more attuned to our digital habits and make conscious choices that support our overall well-being.

In addition to setting boundaries and practicing mindfulness, balancing screen time with offline activities is essential for maintaining a healthy lifestyle. Spending time away from screens allows us to engage in activities that promote physical, mental, and emotional well-being, such as spending time outdoors, exercising, socializing with friends and family, and pursuing hobbies and interests. By incorporating a variety of offline activities into our daily routines, we can reduce reliance on digital devices and create a more balanced and fulfilling life.

Furthermore, incorporating technology breaks and digital detoxes into our routines can help reset our relationship with screens and reduce the negative effects of excessive screen time. This can involve taking short breaks throughout the day to disconnect from screens and engage in activities that promote relaxation and well-being, such as meditation, deep breathing exercises, or simply taking a walk outside. Additionally, scheduling periodic digital detoxes, where we completely disconnect from digital devices for a set period, can provide an opportunity to recharge, reconnect with ourselves and others, and gain perspective on our digital habits.

Moreover, cultivating a supportive digital environment can play a crucial role in managing screen time and promoting overall well-being. This includes surrounding ourselves with people who support and encourage healthy screen habits, as well as creating environments that facilitate mindful and balanced technology use. For example, parents can establish clear rules and expectations around screen time for their children, model healthy screen habits themselves, and create screen-free zones and activities for the whole family to enjoy together. Similarly, workplaces can promote a culture of digital wellness by encouraging employees to take regular breaks from screens, providing opportunities for offline interactions and activities, and offering resources and support for managing digital overload.

Ultimately, managing screen time is essential for maintaining mental health and well-being in the digital age. By setting boundaries, practicing mindful technology use, balancing screen time with offline activities, taking regular technology breaks, and cultivating a supportive digital environment, individuals can reduce the negative effects of excessive screen time and create a healthier relationship with digital technology. By prioritizing our well-being and finding a balance that works for us, we can ensure that screen time enhances rather than detracts from our quality of life in the digital age.

Chapter 5: Building a Healthy Digital Environment

Supporting others in achieving screen serenity involves providing guidance, resources, and encouragement to help individuals develop healthy habits and behaviors around digital technology. One crucial aspect of supporting others in achieving screen serenity is fostering open and honest communication about digital habits and their impact on mental health. By creating a safe space for dialogue, individuals can feel comfortable discussing their struggles with screen time and seeking support and guidance from others. This can involve sharing personal experiences, offering empathy and understanding, and providing practical advice and solutions for managing screen time effectively. Additionally, supporting others in achieving screen serenity requires educating them about the potential risks and consequences of excessive screen time and empowering them to make informed choices about their digital habits. This includes raising awareness of the impact of screen time on mental health, highlighting the importance of setting boundaries and limits, and providing resources and tools for managing screen time effectively.

Furthermore, providing support and encouragement for those struggling with screen time involves helping them identify and address underlying issues that may be contributing to their unhealthy digital habits. This can involve exploring the reasons behind their excessive screen time, such as boredom, stress, loneliness, or a desire for validation, and helping them develop alternative coping strategies and healthier ways of meeting their needs. For example, individuals may benefit from finding alternative ways to cope with stress or boredom, such as engaging in physical activity, practicing mindfulness and relaxation techniques, or pursuing hobbies and interests offline. Additionally, providing social support and connection can help individuals feel less isolated and more empowered to make positive changes in their digital habits. This can involve encouraging them to spend time with friends and family, join support groups or online communities, and engage in meaningful offline activities that promote well-being and fulfillment.

Moreover, supporting others in achieving screen serenity involves modeling healthy screen habits and behaviors ourselves and serving as positive role models for those around us. By demonstrating healthy boundaries around screen time, practicing mindful technology use, and prioritizing offline activities and relationships, we can inspire others to do the same and create a culture of digital wellness in our homes, schools, workplaces, and communities. Additionally, providing encouragement and reinforcement for positive behaviors can help individuals stay motivated and committed to their goals of achieving screen serenity. This can involve celebrating milestones and successes, offering words of encouragement and affirmation, and providing ongoing support and accountability as individuals work towards managing their screen time effectively.

Furthermore, advocating for policies and initiatives that promote digital wellness and support individuals in achieving screen serenity is essential for creating a supportive and empowering environment. This can involve advocating for policies that promote digital literacy and responsible technology use in schools and workplaces, raising awareness of the importance of digital wellness and mental health in public health campaigns and initiatives, and supporting initiatives that provide resources and support for individuals struggling with screen time and digital addiction. By working together to create a culture that values and prioritizes mental health and well-being in the digital age, we can support individuals in achieving screen serenity and ensure that technology enhances rather than detracts from their quality of life.

In conclusion, supporting others in achieving screen serenity involves fostering open and honest communication, providing education and resources, helping individuals identify and address underlying issues, modeling healthy screen habits and behaviors, providing encouragement and reinforcement, and advocating for policies and initiatives that promote digital wellness. By working together to create a supportive and empowering environment, we can help individuals develop healthy habits and behaviors around digital technology and ensure that technology enhances rather than detracts from their mental health and well-being in the digital age.

Chapter 6: Supporting Others in Achieving Screen Serenity

Chapter 6 ventures into the intricate dynamics of community engagement within the digital sphere, unveiling the transformative potency of communal solidarity in navigating the multifaceted landscape of modern digital wellness. Serving as a guiding light, this chapter embarks on an odyssey towards collective empowerment and resilience amidst the ceaseless deluge of digital stimuli. Through a rich tapestry woven from empirical data, personal narratives, and visionary insights, readers embark on a journey through the labyrinth of digital existence, where the force of community emerges as a formidable antidote to the isolating effects of excessive screen time.

This chapter primarily underscores the catalyzing power of communal solidarity—a force transcending individual boundaries and propelling collective action towards a shared vision of digital well-being. Drawing inspiration from historical movements and contemporary grassroots endeavors, the narrative illustrates how collective mobilization can instigate systemic change, from grassroots advocacy campaigns to global initiatives aimed at reshaping the digital landscape. Within the crucible of shared experience, individuals uncover the transformative potential of human connection—a balm for the wounds inflicted by digital disconnection and alienation.

Central to the narrative is the imperative of fostering digital communities rooted in empathy, inclusivity, and ethical integrity—a counterbalance to the pervasive culture of comparison and competition perpetuated by mainstream social media platforms. By nurturing spaces for authentic interaction, meaningful dialogue, and mutual support, communities provide sanctuary from the corrosive effects of digital isolation, nurturing a culture of acceptance and belonging in the digital domain. Whether through online forums, social networking platforms, or community-led initiatives, individuals find solace in digital communities that prioritize human connection over algorithmic engagement metrics, fostering a sense of belonging that transcends temporal and spatial boundaries.

Also, the chapter illuminates the transformative potential of collective advocacy in championing policies and initiatives that promote digital wellness and ethical technology design. From grassroots movements to legislative endeavors, communities wield significant influence in shaping the digital landscape and holding technology conglomerates accountable for their impact on mental health and well-being. Through coordinated action, mobilization of public support, and amplification of marginalized voices, communities catalyze systemic change, paving the way towards a more equitable and humane digital future.

This chapter serves as a clarion call for collective action and community empowerment in the pursuit of digital wellness. Through empathy, resilience, and shared purpose, communities emerge as bastions of support, offering solace, solidarity, and a sense of belonging in an increasingly digitized world. As individuals navigate the complexities of the digital age, the chapter encourages harnessing the power of community to shape a future where technology enriches rather than diminishes human well-being, and where human connection remains paramount in the digital landscape.

8

Chapter 7: Digital Empathy - Nurturing Compassionate Connections in a Virtual World

In the fast-paced, interconnected world we live in, digital technology has redefined how we interact, communicate, and form relationships. While the internet has the power to bring people together from across the globe, it also poses unique challenges to genuine human connection. One of the most profound ways to mitigate these challenges is through cultivating digital empathy—an essential skill in nurturing compassionate and meaningful connections in a virtual world.

Digital empathy refers to the ability to understand and share the feelings of others through digital communication channels. This skill is critical as much of our modern communication happens online, whether through social media, messaging apps, or video calls. Unlike face-to-face interactions, digital communication often lacks the subtle cues of body language and tone, making it harder to convey and interpret emotions accurately. Developing digital empathy can bridge this gap, fostering deeper, more authentic connections.

Empathy in the digital age begins with active listening. In an era where distractions are just a click away, giving someone your full attention can be a powerful act of kindness. When engaging in online conversations, it's important to listen carefully, validate the other person's feelings, and respond thoughtfully. This might involve taking a moment to truly absorb what the other person is saying, rather than hastily typing a response. By doing so, you demonstrate respect and genuine interest, which can significantly enhance the quality of your interactions.

Another crucial aspect of digital empathy is practicing kindness and patience. The anonymity and physical distance of online interactions can sometimes lead to misunderstandings and conflicts. It's easy to forget that there are real people with real feelings on the other side of the screen. When disagreements arise, approach them with a calm and open mind. Take the time to understand the other person's perspective and express your own thoughts respectfully. A little patience and kindness can go a long way in resolving conflicts and building stronger relationships.

Being mindful of the language we use online is also essential. Words can have a powerful impact, especially in the absence of non-verbal cues. Thoughtless or careless comments can easily be misinterpreted and cause unintended harm. To communicate more effectively and empathetically, choose your words carefully. Consider how your message might be received and aim to express yourself in a clear, compassionate manner. Positive language and affirmations can help create a supportive and encouraging online environment.

Creating a safe and inclusive digital space is another key component of digital empathy. This involves being aware of and sensitive to the diverse backgrounds and experiences of others. In group settings, ensure that everyone feels welcome and valued. Encourage open dialogue and respect different viewpoints. By fostering an inclusive atmosphere, you can help build a sense of community and belonging, which is vital for meaningful connections.

Empathy in the digital realm also extends to recognizing and addressing the impact of digital interactions on mental health. It's important to be aware of the potential for online communication to affect someone's emotional well-being. If a friend or colleague seems distressed or withdrawn, reach out and offer support. Sometimes, a simple message of concern or a virtual check-in can make a significant difference. Showing that you care about someone's well-being reinforces trust and strengthens your connection.

Incorporating empathy into our digital interactions requires self-awareness and emotional intelligence. It involves recognizing our own biases and being mindful of how they might influence our online behavior. Take the time to reflect on your digital interactions and consider how you can improve them. This might mean stepping back and thinking about how you would feel if you were in the other person's shoes. By cultivating self-awareness, you can become more attuned to the needs and feelings of others.

Technology can also be leveraged to enhance digital empathy. Video calls, for instance, offer a more personal touch than text messages, allowing for richer communication through facial expressions and tone of voice. When possible, opt for video interactions to foster a deeper connection. Additionally, using emojis and gifs can help convey emotions and add a human element to your messages. While these tools are no substitute for genuine empathy, they can help bridge the emotional gap in digital communication.

Digital empathy is not just about one-on-one interactions; it also involves participating in broader online communities with a compassionate mindset. Contributing positively to online forums, social media groups, or collaborative projects can have a ripple effect, encouraging others to act empathetically as well. Share supportive comments, offer constructive feedback, and celebrate the successes of others. By setting a positive example, you can help cultivate a culture of empathy within your digital circles.

The journey to digital empathy is ongoing, requiring continuous effort and reflection. As our world becomes increasingly digital, the need for empathetic connections grows more crucial. By embracing and practicing digital empathy, we can navigate the virtual landscape with compassion, understanding, and respect. This not only enhances our own well-being but also enriches the lives of those we interact with. In the end, nurturing compassionate connections in a virtual world is about recognizing our shared humanity and striving to make the digital space a more empathetic and connected place for everyone.

Chapter 8: The Role of Social Media in Mental Health

In the digital age, social media has become an integral part of daily life for millions of people worldwide. Platforms like Facebook, Instagram, Twitter, and TikTok provide users with the ability to connect, share, and interact with others on an unprecedented scale. While these platforms offer numerous benefits, such as fostering communication and providing a space for self-expression, they also pose significant challenges to mental health. This chapter delves into the complex relationship between social media and mental health, exploring both its positive and negative impacts, and offering strategies for maintaining a healthy relationship with social media.

The Positive Aspects of Social Media

Social media has revolutionized the way people communicate and connect. For many, these platforms provide a valuable means of staying in touch with friends and family, especially those who live far away. Social media can also serve as a tool for professional networking, enabling individuals to build and maintain business relationships. Additionally, these platforms often provide a sense of community and belonging, especially for those who may feel isolated in their offline lives.

Another positive aspect of social media is its potential to raise awareness about important social issues. Movements such as #MeToo and Black Lives Matter have gained global recognition and support through social media, highlighting the power of these platforms to drive social change. Furthermore, social media can offer support and resources for those struggling with mental health issues, providing a space to share experiences and find solidarity.

The Negative Impacts of Social Media

Despite these benefits, social media can also have detrimental effects on mental health. One of the most significant negative impacts is the phenomenon of comparison culture. On platforms where users often present curated, idealized versions of their lives, it can be easy to fall into the trap of comparing oneself to others. This constant comparison can lead to feelings of inadequacy, low self-esteem, and depression.

Another major concern is the addictive nature of social media. The design of these platforms often encourages continuous engagement, with features such as infinite scrolling and notifications creating a cycle of habitual use. This can lead to excessive screen time, which is associated with a range of mental health issues, including anxiety, depression, and sleep disturbances.

Cyberbullying is another critical issue associated with social media use. The anonymity provided by these platforms can embolden individuals to engage in bullying behavior, leading to significant psychological distress for victims. Additionally, the pressure to maintain a certain image or presence on social media can contribute to stress and anxiety, particularly among younger users.

The Psychological Mechanisms Behind Social Media's Impact

Understanding the psychological mechanisms behind social media's impact on mental health is crucial for developing strategies to mitigate its negative effects. One key mechanism is the role of dopamine, a neurotransmitter associated with pleasure and reward. Social media use, particularly the reception of likes and positive comments, can trigger dopamine release, creating a sense of pleasure and reinforcing the behavior. This reward cycle can contribute to the addictive nature of social media.

Another important factor is the role of social comparison. According to social comparison theory, individuals have a natural tendency to compare themselves to others to evaluate their own abilities and opinions. On social media, where people often share highlights of their lives, these comparisons can lead to negative self-assessments and reduced self-esteem.

Strategies for Healthy Social Media Use

To mitigate the negative effects of social media on mental health, it is essential to develop strategies for healthy use. One effective approach is to set boundaries and limits on social media use. This might involve setting specific times of day for checking social media, using apps that track and limit screen time, or taking regular breaks from social media altogether.

Another important strategy is to curate your social media feed. This means being mindful of who you follow and the type of content you engage with. Following accounts that promote positivity and mental well-being, while unfollowing or muting accounts that contribute to negative feelings, can help create a healthier online environment.

Practicing digital detoxes, where one takes a complete break from social media for a period, can also be beneficial. These breaks can help reset your relationship with social media and provide an opportunity to engage in offline activities that promote well-being, such as spending time in nature, exercising, or pursuing hobbies.

Building Resilience and Digital Literacy

Building resilience and digital literacy is another crucial aspect of maintaining mental health in the age of social media. Digital literacy involves understanding how social media platforms operate, including the ways in which they are designed to capture and hold attention. By becoming more aware of these mechanisms, individuals can make more informed choices about their social media use.

Resilience, on the other hand, involves developing the psychological tools to cope with the challenges posed by social media. This can include practicing mindfulness, developing a strong sense of self-worth independent of social media validation, and seeking support from friends, family, or mental health professionals when needed.

health. By understanding the psychological mechanisms behind its impact and adopting strategies for healthy use, individuals can navigate the digital landscape in a way.

Reflecting on the Role of Social Media

Social media is a double-edged sword, offering both significant benefits and serious challenges to mental health. By understanding the psychological mechanisms behind its impact and adopting strategies for healthy use, individuals can navigate the digital landscape in a way that supports their mental well-being. It is crucial to remain mindful of how social media affects us and to take proactive steps to ensure it serves as a positive force in our lives.

Chapter 9: The Influence of Digital Technology on Different Age Groups

Digital technology permeates every aspect of modern life, affecting people of all ages in unique and profound ways. From toddlers swiping through educational apps to seniors staying connected with loved ones via video calls, the digital revolution has reshaped how we live, learn, and interact. Each age group encounters distinct benefits and challenges when engaging with digital technology, and understanding these nuances is key to fostering healthy, balanced digital habits across the lifespan.

For young children, digital technology offers both incredible opportunities and significant risks. Early childhood is a critical period for brain development, and interactive educational apps and programs can enhance learning by making it engaging and accessible. Children can explore new concepts through gamified learning experiences, developing cognitive and motor skills in the process. However, excessive screen time can interfere with essential developmental activities such as physical play, social interaction, and sleep. Parents and caregivers must strike a balance, ensuring that technology supplements rather than supplants real-world experiences. Setting limits, choosing high-quality content, and co-viewing can help maximize the benefits while minimizing the drawbacks.

Adolescents navigate a complex digital landscape marked by both connectivity and vulnerability. Social media becomes a central part of teenage life, offering a platform for self-expression, connection, and community-building. For many teenagers, online interactions provide a sense of belonging and a way to explore their identities. However, the pressures of social media can also exacerbate insecurities and lead to issues such as cyberbullying, social comparison, and mental health struggles. Teens are particularly susceptible to the lure of digital validation, often measuring their self-worth by the number of likes and followers. Encouraging open communication about online experiences, promoting digital literacy, and teaching critical thinking skills can empower adolescents to navigate these challenges more effectively.

Young adults, often at the forefront of technological adoption, harness digital tools for education, career advancement, and social networking. The transition from adolescence to adulthood is a period of exploration and self-discovery, and digital technology offers myriad resources for personal and professional growth. Online courses and professional networks can provide valuable opportunities for skill development and career progression. However, the omnipresence of digital devices can also lead to distractions, information overload, and burnout. Establishing healthy digital habits, such as time management and mindful usage, is crucial for young adults striving to achieve a balanced and fulfilling life.

Midlife adults, juggling careers, family responsibilities, and social lives, often rely on digital technology for efficiency and convenience. From managing work tasks and household chores to staying connected with family and friends, technology can streamline daily routines and enhance productivity. However, the demands of constant connectivity can contribute to stress and reduce quality time with loved ones. Midlife adults may also face challenges related to digital privacy and security, especially as they engage in online banking, shopping, and personal data management. Prioritizing digital well-being involves setting boundaries, practicing digital detoxes, and staying informed about cybersecurity practices.

For seniors, digital technology can be a lifeline, offering tools to combat isolation and maintain independence. Video calls, social media, and messaging apps allow older adults to stay in touch with family and friends, fostering social connections that are crucial for mental health. Health monitoring devices and telemedicine services can provide significant benefits, enabling seniors to manage health conditions more effectively and access medical care remotely. However, older adults may face barriers to technology adoption, such as a lack of digital literacy or apprehension about new technologies. Providing education and support, designing user-friendly interfaces, and promoting accessible technologies can help seniors embrace the digital world with confidence.

Across all age groups, the influence of digital technology extends beyond individual use, shaping societal norms and behaviors. Families must navigate the complexities of digital interdependence, finding ways to balance screen time with face-to-face interactions. Schools and educators face the challenge of integrating technology into curricula while ensuring that it enhances rather than hinders learning. Workplaces must adapt to the evolving digital landscape, fostering environments that support both productivity and well-being.

To foster a healthy digital environment, it is essential to recognize the unique needs and experiences of each age group. Tailoring strategies to address these differences can help mitigate the negative impacts of digital technology while maximizing its benefits. For young children, this might mean creating tech-free zones and encouraging outdoor play. For adolescents, it could involve promoting digital resilience and online safety. For young adults and midlife adults, it may require developing skills for digital detox and time management. For seniors, offering tech support and designing inclusive technologies can make a significant difference.

The ongoing evolution of digital technology presents both opportunities and challenges. As we move forward, it is crucial to adopt a holistic approach that considers the diverse ways in which technology impacts different age groups. By fostering digital literacy, promoting healthy habits, and supporting intergenerational understanding, we can create a balanced digital ecosystem that enhances well-being and enriches lives across the lifespan. The journey toward digital well-being is a collective effort, requiring empathy, education, and a commitment to nurturing positive, meaningful connections in an increasingly connected world.

11

Chapter 11: Digital Wellness in the Workplace

In today's fast-paced, digitally-driven world, the workplace is a primary arena where technology and mental health intersect. While digital tools have revolutionized how we work, offering unprecedented efficiency and flexibility, they have also introduced new challenges. The constant connectivity can blur the boundaries between work and personal life, leading to stress, burnout, and reduced productivity. Cultivating digital wellness in the workplace is essential for fostering a healthy, productive, and satisfied workforce.

The first step toward digital wellness in the workplace is setting clear boundaries around digital communication. Many employees feel the pressure to be available 24/7, responding to emails and messages even during off-hours. This always-on culture can lead to burnout and decreased job satisfaction. Employers can combat this by establishing policies that respect personal time. For example, instituting no-email policies after certain hours or on weekends can give employees the space they need to recharge. Encouraging employees to set their own boundaries and communicate them to colleagues can also foster a more respectful and balanced digital environment.

Creating tech-free spaces within the workplace can significantly enhance digital wellness. Designating areas where digital devices are discouraged can promote face-to-face interactions, relaxation, and creativity. Break rooms, lounges, and outdoor spaces can serve as tech-free zones where employees can unwind and engage in meaningful conversations without the distraction of screens. These spaces not only provide a mental break but also encourage a sense of community and connection among employees.

Promoting a culture of mindful technology use is crucial. Mindfulness involves being present and fully engaged with whatever one is doing at the moment. When applied to digital technology, it means using devices and applications intentionally rather than out of habit or compulsion. Employers can support mindful technology use by offering training and resources on digital mindfulness practices. Workshops or seminars on managing digital distractions, using technology purposefully, and incorporating mindfulness into daily routines can empower employees to take control of their digital habits.

Regular breaks from screen time are vital for maintaining digital wellness. The Pomodoro Technique, which involves working in focused intervals (typically 25 minutes) followed by short breaks, can help employees manage their time effectively and reduce digital fatigue. Encouraging employees to take short, frequent breaks away from their screens can prevent burnout and boost productivity. Walking meetings or standing desks can also provide physical relief from prolonged sitting and screen exposure.

Digital wellness is not just about managing screen time; it's also about creating a supportive and inclusive work environment. Employers can play a significant role in fostering digital empathy—understanding and responding to the emotional needs of colleagues in digital communications. Promoting a culture of kindness, patience, and understanding in online interactions can enhance team cohesion and overall workplace morale. Providing guidelines for respectful and empathetic digital communication can help employees navigate the challenges of virtual interactions.

Flexible work arrangements, such as remote work and flexible hours, can also contribute to digital wellness. These arrangements offer employees the autonomy to manage their work-life balance more effectively, reducing the stress associated with rigid schedules. However, it's important to provide support and resources for remote employees to ensure they stay connected and engaged. Regular check-ins, virtual team-building activities, and access to mental health resources can help remote workers feel supported and valued.

The role of leadership in promoting digital wellness cannot be over-stated. Leaders set the tone for the organization's culture and practices. By modeling healthy digital habits, such as taking regular breaks, setting boundaries, and practicing digital mindfulness, leaders can inspire their teams to do the same. Openly discussing the importance of digital wellness and providing resources and support can reinforce the organization's commitment to employee well-being.

Implementing digital wellness initiatives requires a holistic approach. Conducting regular assessments of employees' digital habits and wellness needs can provide valuable insights into areas for improvement. Surveys, focus groups, and feedback sessions can help identify specific challenges and opportunities for promoting digital wellness. Based on these insights, organizations can develop tailored strategies and programs that address the unique needs of their workforce.

One effective strategy is to integrate digital wellness into existing wellness programs. Many organizations already offer wellness programs that focus on physical and mental health. Expanding these programs to include digital wellness can provide a more comprehensive approach to employee well-being. Offering resources such as ergonomic assessments, mental health counseling, and workshops on managing digital stress can help employees develop a holistic approach to wellness.

Technology itself can be harnessed to promote digital wellness. There are numerous apps and tools designed to support mindful technology use, manage stress, and enhance productivity. Employers can provide access to these resources as part of their wellness initiatives. For example, apps that track screen time, provide guided meditations, or offer tips for reducing digital distractions can be valuable tools for employees striving to achieve digital balance.

In conclusion, fostering digital wellness in the workplace is essential for creating a healthy, productive, and satisfied workforce. By setting clear boundaries, creating tech-free spaces, promoting mindful technology use, encouraging regular breaks, and supporting flexible work arrangements, employers can help their employees navigate the digital landscape with greater ease and well-being. Leadership plays a crucial role in modeling healthy digital habits and promoting a culture of digital empathy. With a holistic approach that integrates digital wellness into existing wellness programs and leverages technology for support, organizations can cultivate a work environment where employees thrive both online and offline.

12

Chapter 12: Parenting in the Digital Age

Parenting in the digital age presents unique challenges and opportunities. As digital technology becomes an ever-present part of daily life, parents are tasked with guiding their children through a world dominated by screens. From setting appropriate screen time limits to teaching digital citizenship, the role of parents in fostering a balanced and healthy digital environment is more critical than ever. This chapter provides practical advice and strategies for parents to help their children navigate the complexities of digital life.

The first step in managing children's digital lives is understanding the impact of screen time on their development. Excessive screen time has been linked to various negative outcomes, including attention problems, sleep disturbances, and obesity. However, not all screen time is created equal. Educational content and interactive activities can provide meaningful learning experiences, while passive consumption of entertainment media can be less beneficial. Parents need to discern between different types of screen use and set appropriate boundaries.

Setting clear and consistent screen time limits is essential. The American Academy of Pediatrics (AAP) offers guidelines to help parents determine appropriate screen time for different age groups. For children aged 2 to 5, screen time should be limited to one hour per day of high-quality programming. For older children, consistent limits that ensure screens do not interfere with sleep, physical activity, and other essential behaviors are crucial. Creating a family media plan can help establish these boundaries. This plan should outline when, where, and how screens can be used, balancing screen time with other activities.

Modeling healthy digital habits is one of the most powerful tools parents have. Children often emulate the behaviors they observe in their parents. By demonstrating balanced technology use, such as prioritizing face-to-face interactions, setting aside tech-free times, and engaging in offline activities, parents can set a positive example. It is also beneficial for parents to communicate openly with their children about their own screen use, explaining why they set certain limits for themselves and their families.

Choosing quality digital content is another crucial aspect of parenting in the digital age. Parents should seek out age-appropriate, educational, and engaging content that promotes learning and development. Resources like Common Sense Media provide reviews and recommendations for apps, games, and shows that are suitable for children. Co-viewing or co-playing with children can also enhance the educational value of digital content by providing opportunities for discussion and interaction.

Teaching digital citizenship is essential for preparing children to navigate the online world safely and responsibly. Digital citizenship encompasses a range of skills and knowledge, including understanding online privacy, recognizing and avoiding cyberbullying, and practicing respectful online communication. Parents should educate their children about the importance of protecting personal information, recognizing trustworthy sources, and understanding the potential consequences of their online actions. Role-playing different online scenarios can be an effective way to help children learn these concepts.

Online safety is a significant concern for parents. Establishing rules for internet use, such as not sharing personal information, avoiding interactions with strangers, and reporting any inappropriate content or behavior, can help keep children safe. Parents should also familiarize themselves with the privacy settings and parental controls available on devices and platforms their children use. Regularly monitoring their children's online activities and having open conversations about what they encounter online can help parents stay informed and address any issues that arise.

Encouraging offline activities is vital for promoting a balanced lifestyle. Physical activity, creative play, and face-to-face social interactions are crucial for children's development and well-being. Parents should encourage their children to engage in a variety of activities that do not involve screens. Family activities like hiking, board games, and reading can provide quality time together and reduce reliance on digital entertainment. Establishing tech-free zones, such as the dinner table or bedrooms, can also help create spaces for meaningful offline interactions.

Managing digital devices in the home requires setting clear expectations and boundaries. Designating specific times and areas for device use can help prevent overuse and ensure that screens do not interfere with important activities like homework, sleep, and family time. Parents should also consider implementing device-free times, such as during meals and before bedtime, to promote better sleep and strengthen family connections. Consistency is key in enforcing these rules, and involving children in the process of setting these boundaries can help them understand and adhere to them.

Supporting children in developing self-regulation skills is crucial for their long-term digital well-being. Teaching children to recognize their own screen habits and encouraging them to take breaks and engage in other activities can help them develop a healthy relationship with technology. Parents can introduce tools and techniques, such as timers and screen time tracking apps, to help children manage their own screen use. Encouraging children to reflect on how they feel after different types of screen activities can also help them make more mindful choices.

Dealing with resistance and conflicts over screen time is a common challenge for parents. Open communication and negotiation can help address these issues. Parents should explain the reasons behind screen time limits and be willing to listen to their children's perspectives. Compromise and flexibility can be effective in finding solutions that work for the whole family. For example, allowing extra screen time on weekends or as a reward for completing chores can be a way to balance children's desires with healthy limits.

The impact of digital technology on family dynamics is another important consideration. Screens can both connect and isolate family members. While watching a movie together can be a shared experience, individual screen use can lead to isolation. Parents should strive to find a balance between shared and individual screen time, promoting activities that bring the family together. Regular family meetings to discuss screen time rules and address any concerns can help maintain open communication and ensure that everyone's needs are considered.

Understanding the role of social media in children's lives is increasingly important as they grow older. Social media can provide valuable opportunities for social connection and self-expression but also poses risks such as cyberbullying and exposure to inappropriate content. Parents should guide their children in navigating social media by discussing the importance of privacy settings, teaching them to recognize and report harmful behavior, and encouraging them to think critically about the content they share and consume. Being involved and aware of their children's social media activities can help parents provide support and guidance when needed.

The role of schools in supporting digital wellness should not be overlooked. Parents can collaborate with educators to ensure that digital literacy and online safety are part of the school curriculum. Schools can also provide resources and workshops for parents to help them navigate the digital landscape. By working together, parents and schools can create a supportive network that promotes healthy digital habits and addresses any issues that arise.

Finally, it's important for parents to take care of their own digital wellness. Managing their own screen time, setting boundaries, and practicing digital mindfulness can help parents model healthy behaviors for their children. Taking time for self-care and engaging in activities that promote mental and physical well-being can also equip parents with the energy and patience needed to guide their children through the digital age.

In conclusion, parenting in the digital age requires a proactive and informed approach. By setting clear boundaries, modeling healthy habits, choosing quality content, teaching digital citizenship, ensuring online safety, and promoting offline activities, parents can help their children develop a balanced relationship with technology. Open communication, flexibility, and collaboration with schools further enhance this process. As digital technology continues to evolve, parents must remain vigilant and adaptable, equipping themselves and their children with the tools and knowledge needed to thrive in a connected world. Through these efforts, families can achieve screen serenity and foster a harmonious digital environment where everyone can flourish.

13

Chapter 13: Future Trends in Digital Health and Wellness

As technology continues to evolve at a breakneck pace, its impact on our health and wellness is becoming more profound and pervasive. The future promises exciting advancements that could revolutionize the way we manage our mental and physical well-being. In this chapter, we will explore emerging trends and innovations in digital health, examining how they can enhance our lives and what ethical considerations they bring.

The first major trend is the rise of wearable technology. Devices like smartwatches, fitness trackers, and even smart clothing are becoming more sophisticated, offering real-time data on everything from heart rate and sleep patterns to stress levels and blood oxygen saturation. These devices empower individuals to take control of their health by providing actionable insights and personalized recommendations. Imagine a future where your wearable device not only tracks your physical activity but also predicts potential health issues before they become serious, allowing for early intervention and preventative care.

Next, we delve into the burgeoning field of telehealth. The COVID-19 pandemic accelerated the adoption of telehealth services, but its potential extends far beyond the crisis. Telehealth can make healthcare more accessible, especially for those in remote areas or with limited mobility. It enables patients to consult with healthcare providers from the comfort of their homes, reducing the need for travel and wait times. As technology advances, telehealth will become more integrated with other digital health tools, providing a seamless and comprehensive healthcare experience. Virtual reality (VR) and augmented reality (AR) are poised to play a significant role in telehealth, offering immersive therapy sessions and remote diagnostics.

Mental health apps are another game-changer in the digital wellness landscape. These apps provide a range of services, from guided meditations and stress management tools to virtual therapy and support groups. As artificial intelligence (AI) becomes more advanced, mental health apps will offer increasingly personalized and effective interventions. For example, AI-powered chatbots can provide immediate support during a crisis, while machine learning algorithms analyze user data to tailor recommendations for mental wellness activities. The integration of biometric data from wearables with mental health apps will enable a holistic approach to well-being, addressing both physical and mental health needs.

The Internet of Things (IoT) is transforming homes into health-monitoring hubs. Smart home devices can track daily routines, detect unusual patterns, and alert caregivers or medical professionals if something seems amiss. For instance, a smart bed could monitor sleep quality and adjust mattress firmness for optimal rest, while a smart mirror analyzes skin conditions and suggests skincare routines. In the future, our homes could proactively manage our health, providing reminders to take medication, suggesting meal plans based on nutritional needs, and even scheduling doctor's appointments.

Genomic medicine is another exciting frontier in digital health. Advances in DNA sequencing and analysis are making it possible to tailor medical treatments to an individual's genetic makeup. Personalized medicine promises more effective treatments with fewer side effects, as therapies are customized to work with a person's unique genetic profile. This precision approach extends beyond treating illness to preventing it; genetic screening can identify predispositions to certain conditions, enabling proactive measures to maintain health.

The ethical implications of these advancements cannot be overlooked. As we embrace new technologies, we must address issues related to privacy, data security, and equitable access. The vast amount of personal health data generated by wearable devices and smart home systems raises concerns about how this information is stored, shared, and used. Ensuring robust data protection measures and transparent policies is crucial to maintaining trust in digital health innovations.

Equitable access is another critical consideration. While digital health technologies have the potential to democratize healthcare, there is a risk of exacerbating existing disparities if access to these tools is not evenly distributed. Bridging the digital divide by making technology affordable and accessible to all populations is essential for realizing the full benefits of digital health.

One of the most promising aspects of future digital health trends is their potential for early detection and prevention of diseases. AI and machine learning can analyze vast amounts of data to identify subtle patterns and correlations that might be missed by human observation. This capability can lead to earlier diagnosis of conditions like cancer, diabetes, and heart disease, significantly improving treatment outcomes. Preventative healthcare, supported by continuous monitoring and data analysis, can shift the focus from treating illness to maintaining wellness, ultimately reducing healthcare costs and improving quality of life.

The role of big data in healthcare is also set to expand. With the increasing digitization of health records and the proliferation of health-monitoring devices, we are generating an unprecedented amount of health data. Analyzing this data can provide valuable insights into population health trends, identify risk factors for diseases, and inform public health strategies. Collaborative efforts between tech companies, healthcare providers, and researchers will be crucial in harnessing the power of big data for health advancements.

Blockchain technology offers a solution to some of the privacy and security concerns associated with digital health data. By providing a decentralized and secure way to store and share information, blockchain can ensure that health data is tamper-proof and accessible only to authorized individuals. This technology can enhance the transparency and trustworthiness of health data management, paving the way for more widespread adoption of digital health tools.

Looking further into the future, the convergence of biohacking and digital health could lead to unprecedented enhancements in human capabilities. Biohacking involves using science, technology, and self-experimentation to optimize biological functioning. Wearable devices, implantable sensors, and genetic modifications could enable us to enhance physical and cognitive performance, extend lifespan, and improve overall health. While the ethical and societal implications of biohacking are complex and controversial, its potential to revolutionize health and wellness is undeniable.

As digital health technologies evolve, so too will the role of healthcare professionals. The traditional model of healthcare, characterized by periodic visits to a doctor, is giving way to a more continuous and collaborative approach. Healthcare providers will increasingly rely on data from wearable devices, smart home systems, and other digital tools to monitor patients' health in real-time. This shift will require new skills and training for healthcare professionals, as well as changes in healthcare delivery models to integrate digital tools effectively.

The future of digital health also holds exciting possibilities for global health. Mobile health (mHealth) technologies, such as apps and SMS-based health interventions, can reach underserved populations in remote areas, providing access to healthcare information and services. Drones could deliver medical supplies to hard-to-reach locations, and telemedicine can connect patients with specialists anywhere in the world. By leveraging digital health technologies, we can address global health challenges and improve outcomes for populations that have traditionally been underserved.

In conclusion, the future of digital health and wellness is bright, with innovations poised to transform how we manage our well-being. From wearable technology and telehealth to mental health apps and genomic medicine, these advancements offer exciting possibilities for enhancing our health. However, realizing the full potential of these technologies requires addressing ethical considerations, ensuring equitable access, and fostering collaboration between stakeholders. As we navigate this rapidly evolving landscape, staying informed and adaptable will be key to harnessing the benefits of digital health and creating a healthier, more connected world.

14

Conclusion: Embracing the Future with Screen Serenity

As we reach the end of our exploration into the intricate relationship between digital technology and mental health, it's clear that the journey to achieving screen serenity is both complex and profoundly necessary. The digital age, with its myriad of devices and constant connectivity, presents unique challenges and opportunities that require thoughtful navigation and mindful engagement. In this concluding chapter, we will reflect on the key insights from our journey, explore the future of digital wellness, and empower you with the mindset needed to thrive in a connected world.

The digital revolution has fundamentally transformed how we live, work, and interact. From the moment we wake up to the time we go to bed, screens are an integral part of our daily lives. They offer immense benefits, including instant communication, access to vast information, and unprecedented convenience. Yet, these benefits come with a cost. The incessant barrage of notifications, the pressure to stay connected, and the temptation of endless scrolling can lead to digital fatigue, anxiety, and a sense of disconnection from the real world.

Our exploration began with understanding the impact of digital technology on mental health. We delved into how excessive screen time can contribute to issues like anxiety, depression, and sleep disturbances. The key takeaway is that balance is crucial. It's not about demonizing technology but about using it in ways that enhance our lives without compromising our mental well-being. By being mindful of our screen habits and recognizing the signs of digital overload, we can take proactive steps to protect our mental health.

Understanding digital addiction was another critical aspect of our journey. Digital addiction is real and can be as debilitating as other forms of addiction. It manifests in compulsive behaviors, where individuals find it difficult to detach from their devices, leading to negative impacts on their personal and professional lives. Recognizing digital addiction involves self-awareness and honesty about our relationship with technology. Tools like screen time tracking, digital detoxes, and professional support can help individuals regain control and foster healthier digital habits.

The effects of screen time on mental health cannot be overstated. While screens can offer educational and recreational value, excessive use, particularly passive consumption, can lead to physical and mental health issues. We explored strategies for managing screen time, such as setting boundaries, prioritizing offline activities, and creating tech-free zones. These strategies are not just about reducing screen time but about enhancing the quality of our lives by ensuring that technology serves us, not the other way around.

Building a healthy digital environment was another essential topic. This involves creating spaces where technology usage is balanced and purposeful. Encouraging digital empathy and compassionate connections in a virtual world is vital. In an era where online interactions can often be impersonal and harsh, fostering empathy can transform our digital spaces into supportive and positive environments. This requires active listening, respectful communication, and a commitment to understanding others' perspectives.

Supporting others in achieving screen serenity is a communal effort. Whether it's guiding children in the digital age, helping colleagues manage digital stress, or supporting friends and family in finding balance, our collective efforts can make a significant difference. Sharing resources, offering support, and promoting awareness are key components of this endeavor. It's about creating a culture where digital wellness is valued and pursued by everyone.

Looking ahead, the future of digital health and wellness holds exciting possibilities. Advancements in wearable technology, telehealth, mental health apps, and genomic medicine promise to revolutionize how we manage our health. These innovations will offer more personalized and proactive approaches to well-being. However, with these advancements come ethical considerations, particularly around privacy, data security, and equitable access. Ensuring that these technologies benefit everyone requires thoughtful implementation and vigilant oversight.

Embracing screen serenity in the future will also involve staying adaptable and informed. The digital landscape is ever-evolving, and new challenges and opportunities will continue to emerge. By fostering a mindset of continuous learning and adaptability, we can navigate these changes effectively. This involves staying updated on the latest trends, being open to new tools and strategies, and remaining committed to our digital wellness goals.

The role of education in digital wellness cannot be understated. Schools, workplaces, and communities must prioritize digital literacy and well-being. This includes teaching the next generation about responsible technology use, digital citizenship, and the importance of balance. By integrating these principles into educational curricula and workplace training programs, we can build a foundation for a healthier digital future.

Finally, personal responsibility and self-care are at the heart of achieving screen serenity. Each individual has the power to shape their digital experience. This involves setting personal boundaries, being mindful of screen use, and taking time for self-care. Practices like mindfulness meditation, regular physical activity, and engaging in hobbies can counteract the negative effects of excessive screen time. By prioritizing our mental and physical health, we can create a balanced and fulfilling digital life.

In conclusion, the journey to screen serenity is ongoing. It requires awareness, effort, and a willingness to adapt. The digital world offers incredible opportunities, but it also demands that we navigate it thoughtfully and mindfully. By embracing the principles and strategies discussed in this book, we can create a harmonious relationship with technology that enhances our lives and supports our well-being. Together, we can thrive in the digital age, achieving screen serenity and a balanced, connected world.

40

15

Additional Resources: Expanding Your Journey to Screen Serenity

As you continue your journey towards achieving screen serenity and maintaining a balanced relationship with digital technology, having access to a wealth of resources can be invaluable. Below, you'll find a curated list of books, articles, websites, apps, and organizations that provide further insights, tools, and support for managing screen time, fostering digital empathy, and promoting mental well-being in a connected world.

Books

1. **"Digital Minimalism: Choosing a Focused Life in a Noisy World" by Cal Newport**

- Cal Newport offers practical advice on how to reclaim your focus and live a more intentional life by minimizing digital distractions.

1. **"The Shallows: What the Internet Is Doing to Our Brains" by Nicholas Carr**

- Nicholas Carr explores how the internet impacts cognitive processes and provides insights into how we can mitigate its negative effects on our mental health.

1. **"Irresistible: The Rise of Addictive Technology and the Business of Keeping Us Hooked" by Adam Alter**

- Adam Alter examines the addictive nature of modern technology and offers strategies for breaking free from its grip.

1. **"Reclaiming Conversation: The Power of Talk in a Digital Age" by Sherry Turkle**

- Sherry Turkle emphasizes the importance of face-to-face conversation in an increasingly digital world and discusses ways to foster deeper connections.

1. **"Glow Kids: How Screen Addiction Is Hijacking Our Kids – and How to Break the Trance" by Nicholas Kardaras**

- Nicholas Kardaras delves into the impact of screen addiction on children and offers guidance for parents to help their kids develop healthy digital habits.

Articles and Research Papers

1. **"The Impact of Digital Screen Time on Mental Health" - American Psychological Association**

- This article provides an overview of the current research on the effects of screen time on mental health and offers recommendations for managing screen use.

1. **"Social Media Use and Perceived Social Isolation Among Young Adults in the U.S." - Journal of Preventive Medicine**

· This research paper explores the link between social media use and feelings of social isolation, offering insights into how to mitigate negative effects.

1. **"Understanding the Role of Digital Empathy in Online Interactions" - International Journal of Human-Computer Interaction**

· This paper examines the concept of digital empathy and its importance in fostering positive online interactions.

1. **"The Effects of Digital Technology on Children's Mental Health" - UNICEF**

· UNICEF's comprehensive report on the impact of digital technology on children's mental health and development.

1. **"The Role of Mindfulness in Reducing the Negative Effects of Screen Time" - Mindfulness Journal**

· An exploration of how mindfulness practices can help counteract the adverse effects of excessive screen time.

Websites and Online Resources

1. **Common Sense Media (www.commonsensemedia.org)**

- Provides reviews and advice on media and technology for families, helping parents make informed decisions about their children's digital consumption.

1. **Center for Humane Technology (www.humanetech.com)**

- Offers resources and strategies for creating technology that aligns with human well-being and ethical values.

1. **Digital Wellbeing (wellbeing.google)**

- Google's initiative provides tools and tips for managing screen time and promoting digital wellness.

1. **Mindful Techie (www.mindfultechie.com)**

- Offers workshops and resources on integrating mindfulness with technology use to create a more balanced digital life.

1. **Headspace (www.headspace.com)**

- A mindfulness and meditation app that includes features designed to help manage screen time and reduce digital stress.

Apps and Tools

1. **Moment**

- An app that tracks your screen time and provides insights and tools to help you reduce your phone usage and focus on what's important.

1. **Forest**

- This app encourages you to stay focused by planting virtual trees that grow when you avoid using your phone.

1. **Freedom**

- A productivity app that blocks distracting websites and apps, helping you stay focused and productive.

1. **Calm**

- Offers guided meditations, sleep stories, and mindfulness programs that can help mitigate the stress and anxiety associated with digital overload.

1. **RescueTime**

- Tracks your digital activity to help you understand how you spend your time and make more informed decisions about your screen use.

Organizations

1. **The National Institute of Mental Health (NIMH)**

- Provides resources and research on the effects of digital technology on mental health, offering guidance for managing screen time.

1. **Mental Health America (MHA)**

- Offers resources and support for mental health issues, including those related to digital technology and screen time.

1. **The American Academy of Pediatrics (AAP)**

- Provides guidelines and resources for parents on managing children's screen time and promoting healthy digital habits.

1. **The Anxiety and Depression Association of America (ADAA)**

- Offers resources and support for anxiety and depression, including the impact of digital technology on mental health.

1. **The Digital Wellness Collective**

- A network of experts and organizations dedicated to promoting digital wellness and creating a healthier relationship with technology.

By leveraging these resources, you can continue to explore and implement strategies for achieving screen serenity. Each resource offers unique insights and practical advice to help you navigate the digital landscape mindfully and compassionately. As you move forward, remember that achieving balance is a continuous journey, one that requires ongoing effort, reflection, and support. Embrace the tools and knowledge available to you, and take proactive steps to create a healthier, more fulfilling relationship with digital technology.